THE PHILOSOPHY OF SHORINJI KEMPO

A Journey Towards Mastery: From Basic Principles to Advanced Techniques

KAMERON JALEN

Table of Contents

Introduction

Shorinji Kempo is a form of martial art that originated in Japan and incorporates many techniques for self-defense, physical fitness, and a philosophical approach to the development of the individual. Founded in the late 1940s by Doshin So, a former soldier and martial artist, Shorinji Kempo draws influence from a variety of ancient martial arts, primarily Chinese Shaolin Kung Fu, and places an emphasis on training that takes a holistic approach.

Key Features of Shorinji Kempo:

• **Techniques**: The art includes strikes, kicks, joint locks, throws, and grappling techniques, allowing practitioners to defend themselves against various attacks.

• **Philosophy**: Shorinji Kempo emphasizes self-improvement, mutual respect, and the importance of community. It integrates physical training with mental and spiritual growth, promoting values such as humility, perseverance, and compassion.

• **Training**: Classes typically involve a combination of solo and partner drills, kata (pre-arranged forms), and free practice (randori). Students also learn about the history and philosophy of the art, making the training well-rounded.

• **Uniform and Ranking**: Practitioners wear a distinctive uniform called a "karategi," often adorned with a belt indicating their rank. The ranking system helps motivate students and provides a clear progression path.

• **Global Reach**: Since its inception, Shorinji Kempo has spread internationally, with numerous dojos (training halls) established around the world. The organization focuses on fostering a sense of community among its practitioners, regardless of geographical location.

• **Physical and Mental Benefits**: Practicing Shorinji Kempo can improve physical fitness, flexibility, coordination, and self-defense skills. It also promotes mental clarity, focus, and emotional balance, making it beneficial for overall well-being.

Shorinji Kempo is not just a martial art but a comprehensive system for personal development that encourages practitioners to grow physically, mentally, and socially while fostering a sense of community and mutual support.

CHAPTER 1: THE PHILOSOPHY OF SHORINJI KEMPO

The Philosophy Behind Shorinji Kempo

The philosophy behind Shorinji Kempo is deeply rooted in the principles of personal development, mutual respect, and the promotion of peace. Here are the key elements of its philosophy:

1. Self-Improvement: At its core, Shorinji Kempo emphasizes the importance of self-discovery and personal growth. Practitioners are encouraged to strive for their best selves through disciplined training, reflection, and mindfulness. This journey is not only about mastering physical techniques but also about cultivating mental and emotional resilience.

2. Mutual Respect: Shorinji Kempo teaches the value of respect for oneself and others. Practitioners learn to appreciate the strengths and weaknesses of their training partners, fostering an environment of cooperation rather than competition. This mutual respect extends beyond the dojo, promoting harmony within the community and society.

3. Balance of Body and Mind: The philosophy advocates for a holistic approach to training, where physical conditioning is complemented by mental and spiritual development. Practitioners learn to harmonize their physical abilities with mental focus, creating a balanced and integrated approach to self-defense and personal growth.

4. Compassion and Altruism: Doshin So, the founder of Shorinji Kempo, believed in the importance of using martial arts to promote peace and protect the weak. The philosophy encourages practitioners to develop compassion and a sense of responsibility toward others, motivating them to use their skills for the greater good rather than for aggression or self-interest.

5. Community and Global Awareness: Shorinji Kempo promotes a sense of community among its practitioners. The art transcends cultural and geographical boundaries, encouraging students to connect with others and share their experiences. This global perspective fosters understanding and cooperation among diverse groups.

6. Mindfulness and Presence: Practitioners are taught to cultivate mindfulness, being fully present during training and in daily life. This focus enhances their ability to respond to challenges effectively, both on and off the mat.

7. **Philosophical Teachings**: Shorinji Kempo incorporates teachings from various philosophical traditions, including Zen Buddhism. These teachings emphasize the importance of meditation, reflection, and understanding the nature of self and existence.

The philosophy of Shorinji Kempo is not merely about physical combat skills; it is a comprehensive framework for personal development that integrates mind, body, and spirit. By promoting values of respect, compassion, and community, Shorinji Kempo aims to create individuals who are not only proficient in martial arts but also contribute positively to society.

Core Principles And Values

The core principles and values of Shorinji Kempo serve as the foundation for its practice and philosophy, guiding practitioners in their training and interactions. Here are the main principles:

1. Mutual Assistance: Shorinji Kempo promotes the idea that practitioners should support each other in their training journeys. This principle fosters a sense of community and teamwork, emphasizing that growth comes from collaboration rather than competition.

2. Respect: Respect is a fundamental value in Shorinji Kempo, extending to oneself, training partners, instructors, and the art itself. Practitioners are taught to honor the efforts and achievements of others, creating a positive and nurturing training environment.

3. Self-Discipline: Self-discipline is crucial for personal growth in Shorinji Kempo.

Practitioners are encouraged to cultivate discipline in their training, enabling them to overcome challenges, improve their skills, and maintain a consistent practice.

4. Perseverance: The value of perseverance is emphasized as practitioners encounter difficulties and setbacks. Shorinji Kempo teaches that persistence in the face of adversity is essential for achieving mastery and personal development.

5. Compassion and Altruism: Practitioners are encouraged to develop compassion for others and use their skills to protect and assist those in need. This value reflects the belief that martial arts should be used for peace and the betterment of society, rather than for aggression or personal gain.

6. Balance: Shorinji Kempo promotes the importance of balance—between physical strength and mental focus, individual needs and community responsibilities, and self-defense and peaceful resolution. Practitioners learn to harmonize these elements in their lives and training.

7. Mindfulness: Mindfulness is a key aspect of Shorinji Kempo, with an emphasis on being present in the moment during training and daily life. Practitioners learn to cultivate awareness and focus, enhancing their ability to respond effectively to challenges.

8. Continuous Learning: The pursuit of knowledge and understanding is encouraged in Shorinji Kempo. Practitioners are taught that learning is a lifelong journey, both within the martial art and in broader life experiences. This value emphasizes humility and the willingness to grow.

9.   Philosophical   Understanding: Practitioners are encouraged to explore the philosophical teachings underlying Shorinji Kempo, incorporating insights from various traditions to deepen their understanding of themselves and their place in the world.

These core principles and values form the heart of Shorinji Kempo, guiding practitioners in their training and helping them develop not only as martial artists but as compassionate, respectful individuals. Through the integration of these values, Shorinji Kempo aims to cultivate a sense of community and promote peace in society.

The evolution of Shorinji Kempo reflects a dynamic blend of traditional martial arts, modern training methods, and a strong philosophical foundation. Its growth from a local Japanese practice to a global community underscores its enduring appeal and relevance in contemporary society. Through its commitment to personal development and ethical principles, Shorinji Kempo remains a holistic martial art that continues to inspire practitioners around the world.

The Concept Of "Kenshi" (Warrior)

The concept of "kenshi" (剣士) in Shorinji Kempo and Japanese martial arts refers to a warrior or practitioner who embodies not only physical skills but also a deep understanding of the philosophical and ethical dimensions of martial arts. Here are the key aspects of the kenshi concept:

1. Definition of Kenshi: The term "kenshi" literally translates to "sword person" or "sword master" in Japanese. In the context of Shorinji Kempo, it represents someone who has trained extensively in martial arts and has developed both technical proficiency and a warrior's mindset.

2. Physical Proficiency: A kenshi is expected to demonstrate a high level of physical skill, including striking, grappling, and self-defense techniques. This proficiency is developed through rigorous training, including kata (forms), randori (free practice), and sparring.

3. Mental and Emotional Strength: Beyond physical ability, a kenshi is characterized by mental resilience and emotional balance. Training fosters qualities such as focus, discipline, perseverance, and the ability to remain calm under pressure. These traits are essential for effective self-defense and personal growth.

4. Philosophical Understanding: Kenshi are encouraged to delve into the philosophical teachings of Shorinji Kempo, including concepts of mindfulness, respect, and the interconnectedness of all beings. This understanding informs their approach to training and life, emphasizing that martial arts is as much about the mind and spirit as it is about physical combat.

5. Ethics and Responsibility: A kenshi carries the ethical responsibility to use their skills for good. This includes protecting the vulnerable, promoting peace, and embodying values such as compassion and mutual respect. Kenshi are taught that martial arts should never be used for aggression or personal gain.

6. Continuous Learning: The journey of a kenshi is one of lifelong learning. Practitioners are encouraged to remain humble and open to new experiences, recognizing that mastery is a continuous process. This attitude fosters growth both within martial arts and in other aspects of life.

7. Community and Mutual Support: Kenshi are part of a larger community of practitioners. They are expected to support and uplift their peers, fostering a sense of camaraderie and collective growth. This mutual assistance enhances the training experience and reinforces the values of respect and cooperation.

8. Cultural Heritage: The role of the kenshi is deeply rooted in Japan's martial arts culture, reflecting historical traditions of the samurai and warrior ethos. This heritage informs the practice of Shorinji Kempo, connecting modern practitioners to a rich lineage of martial arts.

The concept of kenshi in Shorinji Kempo embodies a holistic approach to martial arts training that integrates physical skills, mental resilience, ethical responsibility, and community support. Kenshi are not just skilled fighters but well-rounded individuals committed to personal development and the betterment of society. This comprehensive view of the warrior spirit enriches the practice of Shorinji Kempo and inspires practitioners to strive for excellence in all areas of their lives.

The spiritual and ethical aspects of Shorinji Kempo are integral to its practice, shaping practitioners into well-rounded individuals who strive for personal growth and contribute positively to society. By fostering mindfulness, compassion, and a sense of responsibility, Shorinji Kempo promotes not only effective self-defense skills but also a holistic approach to life that enhances the well-being of individuals and their communities.

CHAPTER 2
Stances And Footwork

In Shorinji Kempo, stances and footwork are foundational components that contribute to effective movement, balance, and power in techniques. Understanding these elements is crucial for practitioners to develop their skills and execute techniques effectively. Here's an overview of the key stances and footwork used in Shorinji Kempo:

<u>Key Stances</u>

Kiba Dachi (Horse Stance):

• **Description**: A wide stance with feet parallel and shoulder-width apart, knees bent, and the body lowered.

• **Purpose**: Provides a stable base for strikes and techniques, enhancing balance and strength. It is often used in training to develop leg strength and stability.

Zenkutsu Dachi (Forward Stance):

• **Description**: A long stance with one foot forward and the back leg straight, creating a stable triangular base.

• **Purpose**: Used for delivering powerful forward strikes and maintaining balance while moving. This stance allows for greater reach and weight distribution.

Kukutsu Dachi (Back Stance):

• **Description**: A stance with most of the weight on the back leg, with the front leg slightly bent and positioned forward.

• **Purpose**: Provides stability and readiness for defensive techniques. It allows practitioners to quickly react and shift weight when countering attacks.

Neko Ashi Dachi (Cat Stance):

• **Description**: A low stance where most of the weight is on the back foot, while the front foot is lightly touching the ground.

• **Purpose**: Enhances mobility and enables quick movement while maintaining a low center of gravity. This stance is often used for deceptive movements and counters.

Shiko Dachi (Square Stance):

• **Description**: A stance with feet turned outward, knees bent, and the body lowered.

• **Purpose**: Provides a strong base for lateral movements and defensive techniques. It allows practitioners to shift their weight easily and respond to attacks from different angles.

<u>**Footwork Techniques:**</u>

- **Step and Slide**: Practitioners learn to move by stepping and sliding their feet, maintaining balance and control. This technique is essential for closing distance, evading attacks, or repositioning for strikes.

- **Cross Step**: This movement involves crossing one foot over the other to change angles quickly. It allows for evasive movements or positioning for counterattacks while maintaining a low stance.

- **Lateral Movement**: Practitioners are trained to move sideways while maintaining their stances, enabling them to evade attacks and create advantageous angles for countering.

- **Pivoting**: Pivoting on the ball of the foot allows practitioners to change direction quickly without losing balance. This technique is crucial for avoiding strikes and positioning for counters.

• **Back Stepping**: Practitioners learn to step back while maintaining their stance, allowing them to create distance from an opponent or evade incoming attacks effectively.

Stances and footwork are vital elements of Shorinji Kempo that contribute to a practitioner's effectiveness in techniques, balance, and overall martial arts proficiency. Mastering these components allows students to execute strikes, defenses, and transitions fluidly while maintaining control and stability. Through dedicated practice, practitioners develop a strong foundation that enhances their performance in both training and self-defense scenarios.

Basic Techniques (Kihon)

In Shorinji Kempo, "kihon" refers to the fundamental techniques that form the foundation of the martial art. Mastering these basic techniques is essential for building a strong skill set and developing proficiency in more advanced techniques. Here's an overview of the basic techniques commonly taught in Shorinji Kempo:

1. Strikes (Atemi):

- **Gyaku Zuki (Reverse Punch)** A powerful punch delivered with the rear hand, emphasizing hip rotation for added strength.

- **Oi Zuki (Lunge Punch)** A forward punch using the leading hand while stepping forward, promoting momentum and reach.

- **Mae Geri (Front Kick)**

A straight kick delivered with the front foot, targeting the opponent's midsection or face.

- **Yoko Geri (Side Kick)**

A side kick executed by extending the leg sideways, aimed at the opponent's torso or head.

- **Ushiro Geri (Back Kick)**

A kick delivered by thrusting the leg backward, often used to counter an attack from behind.

2. Blocks (Uke):

- **Jodan Uke (High Block)**

A defensive block aimed at protecting the head from high attacks, executed with the forearm.

- **Chudan Uke (Middle Block)**

A block directed at the midsection, used to

defend against punches or strikes aimed at the torso.

- **Gedan Barai (Low Block)** A low block to protect against low attacks, sweeping the arm across the body to deflect strikes.

3. Kicks (Geri):

- **Ashi Barai (Foot Sweep)** A technique used to sweep an opponent's foot to destabilize them, often executed while stepping to the side.

- **Kansetsu Geri (Joint Kick)** A targeted kick aimed at the opponent's joints, such as the knees, to cause pain and disrupt balance.

4. Joint Locks (Kansetsu Waza):

• **Kote Gaeshi (Wrist Lock)**
A technique used to control an opponent's wrist, often applied when defending against a grab or strike.

• **Ude Hishigi (Arm Lock)**
A joint lock applied to the arm, typically executed while grappling or countering an attack.

5. Throws (Nage Waza):

• **O Soto Gari (Major Outer Reap)**
A throwing technique where the practitioner uses their body to sweep the opponent's leg, causing them to fall.

• **Ippon Seoi Nage (One-Arm Shoulder Throw)**
A shoulder throw executed by gripping the

opponent's arm and using body momentum to throw them over the shoulder.

6. Movement Techniques:

- **Tai Sabaki (Body Movement)** The practice of moving the body to evade attacks or create angles for counterattacks. Effective tai sabaki is essential for both offense and defense.

- **Hiki Ashi (Pulling Feet)** A technique used to retreat while maintaining a low stance, allowing for quick movement and readiness for counterattacks.

The basic techniques (kihon) of Shorinji Kempo provide the essential skills necessary for effective self-defense and martial arts practice. By mastering these techniques, practitioners develop a strong foundation that allows them to progress to more advanced skills and applications. Consistent practice of kihon is crucial for building strength, coordination, and confidence, enabling students to grow in their martial arts journey.

Striking Techniques (Tsuki)

In Shorinji Kempo, striking techniques, known as "tsuki," are fundamental for effective self-defense and combat. These techniques focus on delivering powerful, precise strikes while maintaining balance and control. Here's an overview of the primary striking techniques taught in Shorinji Kempo:

1. Gyaku Zuki (Reverse Punch):

• **Description**: A powerful punch delivered with the rear hand while rotating the hips for added force.

Execution:

• Start in a forward stance (zenkutsu dachi).

• Rotate the hips and shoulders as you extend the rear arm forward to strike.

• Keep the other hand in a guarding position.

2. Oi Zuki (Lunge Punch):

• **Description**: A forward punch delivered with the leading hand while stepping forward to close distance.

Execution:

• Begin in a guard position.

• Step forward with the front foot while simultaneously extending the front arm to punch.

• Ensure proper weight transfer for power.

3. Kizami Zuki (Jab):

- **Description**: A quick, straight punch delivered with the lead hand.

Execution:

- Start in a guard position with hands up.

- Extend the lead arm quickly while keeping the other hand in a guarding position.

- Retract immediately to maintain defense.

4. Tate Zuki (Vertical Punch):

- **Description**: A punch delivered with a vertical fist, often targeting the chin or jaw.

Execution:

- Begin in a guard position.

- Rotate the arm so that the fist is vertical as you punch forward.

- Use hip rotation for added power.

5. Shuto Uchi (Knife Hand Strike):

• **Description**: A strike delivered with the edge of the hand, targeting vulnerable areas like the neck or temple.

Execution:

• Start in a guard position.

• Extend the arm with a downward motion, keeping the fingers together and hand relaxed.

• Aim for the target with the edge of the hand.

6. Uraken (Back Fist Strike):

• **Description**: A quick, horizontal strike delivered with the back of the fist, often targeting the opponent's face.

Execution:

• Begin in a guard position.

• Rotate the wrist as you extend the arm, striking with the back of the fist.

• Maintain balance and control throughout the movement.

7. Mune Tsuki (Chest Punch):

• **Description**: A punch directed at the opponent's torso, often used in combination with other techniques.

Execution:

• Start in a guard position.

• Step forward and deliver a punch targeting the midsection.

• Focus on generating power from the legs and hips.

8. Atemi (Striking Techniques):

• **Description**: General term for various striking techniques used to distract or incapacitate an opponent.

Execution:

• Involves a combination of punches, kicks, and open-hand strikes.

• Use quick, powerful strikes to create openings for further techniques.

Key Principles of Striking Techniques:

• **Hip Rotation**: Effective strikes rely on proper hip and shoulder rotation to generate power. Engage the core for maximum strength.

• **Breathing**: Coordinating breathing with strikes helps maintain energy and focus. Exhale sharply upon impact to enhance power.

• **Targeting**: Striking techniques should be aimed at vulnerable areas of the opponent's body (e.g., head, throat, solar plexus) for maximum effectiveness.

• **Distance Management**: Understanding distance is crucial for effective striking. Maintain proper spacing to ensure strikes land while minimizing vulnerability to counters.

The striking techniques (tsuki) in Shorinji Kempo are essential for developing effective self-defense skills and enhancing overall martial arts proficiency. By mastering these techniques, practitioners improve their power, speed, and accuracy, contributing to their growth as well-rounded martial artists. Regular practice of striking techniques is vital for building confidence and competence in real-world situations.

Kicking Techniques (Geri)

In Shorinji Kempo, kicking techniques, referred to as "geri," are integral to a practitioner's arsenal. Kicks provide powerful offensive options and can be used defensively to maintain distance or disrupt an opponent's balance. Here's an overview of the primary kicking techniques taught in Shorinji Kempo:

1. Mae Geri (Front Kick):

• **Description**: A straightforward kick aimed at the opponent's torso or face, delivered with the front foot.

Execution:

• Start in a guard position with feet shoulder-width apart.

• Lift the knee and extend the foot forward, striking with the ball of the foot or the instep.

• Retract the leg quickly to return to the guard position.

2. Yoko Geri (Side Kick):

• **Description**: A lateral kick aimed at the opponent's midsection or head, using the heel or the edge of the foot.

Execution:

• Begin in a guard position.

• Pivot on the supporting foot while lifting the knee and extending the kicking leg sideways.

• Strike with the heel or the edge of the foot and retract quickly.

3. Ushiro Geri (Back Kick):

• **Description**: A powerful kick delivered by thrusting the leg backward, targeting an opponent behind you.

Execution:

• Start in a guard position.

• Shift your weight onto the supporting leg while kicking the back leg straight back, aiming to strike with the heel.

• Keep your head and upper body upright for balance and control.

4. Mawashi Geri (Roundhouse Kick):

• **Description**: A circular kick aimed at the opponent's head or torso, striking with the shin or instep.

Execution:

• Begin in a guard position.

• Pivot on the supporting foot while bringing the knee up and then extending the leg in a circular motion.

• Aim to strike with the shin or instep, retracting the leg quickly after impact.

5. Kaiten Geri (Turning Kick):

• **Description**: A kick delivered by rotating the body and striking with the heel or the edge of the foot, often used to surprise an opponent.

Execution:

• Start in a guard position.

• Pivot on the supporting foot and turn your body while lifting the kicking leg.

• Extend the leg in a turning motion to strike the target.

6. Tobi Geri (Jumping Kick):

• **Description**: A dynamic kick executed while jumping, aimed at the opponent's head or upper body.

Execution:

• Start in a guard position.

• Jump off the back foot while extending the kicking leg.

• Aim for a high target, landing safely and maintaining balance upon return.

7. Gedan Geri (Low Kick):

• **Description**: A kick aimed at the opponent's lower body, such as the knee or thigh, often used to disrupt balance.

Execution:

• Begin in a guard position.

• Lift the knee and extend the foot low, striking with the ball of the foot or shin.

• Quickly retract to avoid counterattacks.

<u>**Key Principles of Kicking Techniques:**</u>

• **Balance and Stability**: Maintaining balance is essential for effective kicking. Proper stance and core engagement help ensure stability during kicks.

• **Hip Movement**: Engage the hips during kicks to generate power. Rotating the hips adds strength and momentum to the strike.

• **Targeting**: Aim for vulnerable areas of the opponent's body to maximize the effectiveness of kicks. Kicking high or low can create openings for further techniques.

• **Follow-through and Retraction**: After executing a kick, quickly retract the leg to return to a defensive position. This readiness allows for immediate follow-up techniques or defense.

• **Breath Control**: Coordinating breath with kicks can enhance power and focus. Exhale sharply upon impact to maximize the effectiveness of the kick.

Kicking techniques (geri) in Shorinji Kempo are essential for developing versatility and effectiveness in self-defense situations. By mastering these techniques, practitioners can improve their striking power, speed, and precision, contributing to their overall growth as martial artists. Regular practice of kicking techniques is crucial for building confidence and competence in both training and real-world applications.

Grappling Techniques (Nage And Osaekomi)

In Shorinji Kempo, grappling techniques, known as "nage" (throwing) and "osaekomi" (holding or pinning), play a significant role in self-defense and combat strategy. These techniques focus on controlling an opponent through leverage, balance, and body mechanics. Here's an overview of the primary grappling techniques taught in Shorinji Kempo:

Nage Techniques (Throwing Techniques)

O Soto Gari (Major Outer Reap):

- **Description**: A powerful throw that involves sweeping the opponent's leg from the outside while using body weight to off-balance them.

Execution:

- Approach your opponent and grip their collar or shoulder.

- Step to the side, planting your foot beside their foot.

• Use your body weight to sweep their leg while pulling them forward and down.

Ippon Seoi Nage (One-Arm Shoulder Throw):

• **Description**: A shoulder throw where the practitioner uses one arm to lift and throw the opponent over their shoulder.

Execution:

• Grip the opponent's arm while stepping forward.

• Turn your back to them, dropping your center of gravity.

• Use your hips and legs to lift and throw them over your shoulder.

Koshi Nage (Hip Throw):

• **Description**: A throw that involves using the hips to lift and throw the opponent.

Execution:

• Secure a grip on your opponent's collar or waist.

• Step close, turning your body so your hip is aligned with theirs.

• Drop your center of gravity and lift them over your hip to throw them.

Tai Otoshi (Body Drop):

• **Description**: A technique that involves dropping the body while pulling the opponent down and sideways.

Execution:

• Begin by grasping your opponent's arm.

• Step forward and to the side, dropping your weight and pulling them down across your body.

• Use your hip and shoulder to help guide their fall.

Kake Nage (Hooking Throw):

• **Description**: A throw that utilizes a hooking motion to off-balance and throw the opponent.

Execution:

• Get into close range and grab your opponent's arm.

• Use a circular motion to pull them off balance while stepping sideways.

• Complete the throw by using your hip or shoulder for leverage.

• Osaekomi Techniques (Holding/Pinning Techniques)

Kuzushi (Breaking Balance):

• **Description**: The principle of off-balancing an opponent to set up throws or pins.

Execution:

• Apply pressure or leverage to the opponent's body, causing them to lose their balance.

• Use footwork and body movement to create openings for throws or pins.

Kesa Gatame (Scarf Hold):

• **Description**: A pinning technique where the practitioner wraps an arm around the opponent's head and controls their body.

Execution:

• Move into position beside the opponent, securing their head with one arm.

• Use your other arm to grip their wrist or control their body.

• Keep your weight distributed over them to maintain control.

Tate Shiho Gatame (Vertical Four-Quarter Hold):

• **Description**: A pin where the practitioner holds the opponent's shoulders down while controlling their body.

Execution:

• Position yourself above the opponent, straddling their body.

• Use your hands to push down on their shoulders while controlling their hips or legs.

• Maintain pressure to keep them pinned.

Yoko Shiho Gatame (Horizontal Four-Quarter Hold):

• **Description**: A pin that involves holding the opponent's shoulders while lying perpendicular to their body.

Execution:

• Position yourself alongside the opponent, lying across their body.

• Use your arms to pin their shoulders down while controlling their hips or legs.

• Keep your weight balanced to maintain the hold.

Ude Hishigi (Arm Lock):

• **Description**: A technique that applies pressure to the opponent's arm joint, often used during grappling.

Execution:

• As you secure a hold, position your body to control the opponent's arm.

• Apply pressure to the elbow or wrist joint, forcing the opponent to submit or lose balance.

Key Principles of Grappling Techniques:

- **Balance and Leverage**: Effective grappling relies on understanding balance and using leverage to control the opponent. Practitioners should focus on maintaining their balance while disrupting their opponent's.

- **Body Mechanics**: Utilizing body weight and mechanics is essential for executing throws and holds effectively. Proper posture and body alignment enhance control and power.

- **Breath Control**: Coordinating breath with grappling movements can help maintain focus and energy. Breathing deeply during exertion can aid in relaxation and stability.

- **Adaptability**: Grappling techniques often require adaptability to different situations.

Practitioners should be prepared to adjust their techniques based on the opponent's reactions.

Grappling techniques (nage and osaekomi) in Shorinji Kempo are vital for developing control, balance, and effective self-defense skills. By mastering these techniques, practitioners enhance their ability to manage confrontations through throws and pins, making them versatile martial artists. Regular practice of grappling techniques is essential for building confidence and competence in both training and real-world applications.

Advanced Techniques And Variations

In Shorinji Kempo, advanced techniques build upon the foundational skills learned through basic and intermediate training. These techniques often involve a combination of strikes, throws, locks, and counters, requiring practitioners to have a solid understanding of body mechanics, timing, and adaptability. Here's an overview of some advanced techniques and variations commonly practiced in Shorinji Kempo:

1. Advanced Striking Techniques

Jodan Mawashi Geri (High Roundhouse Kick):

• **Description**: An elevated roundhouse kick aimed at the opponent's head or upper body, utilizing hip rotation for added power.

• **Variation**: **Ura Mawashi Geri (Reverse Roundhouse Kick)**, where the kick is delivered in a reverse motion, targeting the opponent's head from behind.

Tobi Zuki (Jumping Punch):

• **Description**: A powerful punch executed while jumping, aimed at catching the opponent off guard.

• **Variation**: **Tobi Mae Geri (Jumping Front Kick)**, where the practitioner jumps and delivers a front kick instead.

2. Advanced Kicking Techniques

Nidan Geri (Jumping Front Kick):

• **Description**: A high front kick executed from a jump, targeting the opponent's face or chest.

- **Variation**: **Mune Geri (Chest Kick)**, where the kick is aimed specifically at the opponent's chest.

Kage Geri (Crescent Kick):

- **Description**: A circular kick that strikes with the inside edge of the foot, targeting the opponent's head or torso.

- **Variation**: **Ushiro Kage Geri (Back Crescent Kick)**, where the kick is delivered backward in a crescent motion.

3. Advanced Grappling Techniques

Ashi Guruma (Leg Wheel):

- **Description**: A throwing technique that involves using the opponent's leg to destabilize and throw them.

Execution:

• Approach the opponent and secure a grip on their body.

• Sweep one of their legs while using your body weight to off-balance them, completing the throw.

Hiki Otoshi (Pulling Drop):

• **Description**: A technique that involves pulling the opponent while simultaneously dropping your body weight, causing them to fall.

Execution:

• Secure a grip on the opponent's collar or arm.

• Pull them toward you while dropping your body to create a throwing effect.

4. Advanced Joint Locks and Control Techniques

Kansetsu Nage (Joint Throw):

• **Description**: A technique that combines throwing with joint locks, applying pressure to force the opponent to the ground.

Execution: Secure a hold on the opponent's arm and execute a throw while maintaining the lock.

Ude Garami (Arm Entanglement)

• **Description**: A complex joint lock involving entangling the opponent's arm, often leading to a throw or submission.

Execution: Use body positioning to entangle the opponent's arm while controlling their balance and positioning.

5. Combination Techniques

Tsuki to Geri Combination (Punch to Kick):

• **Description**: A series of techniques that combine strikes and kicks fluidly to overwhelm the opponent.

Execution: Start with a punch (gyaku zuki) followed immediately by a kick (mae geri), maintaining fluidity and speed.

Throw to Lock Combination:

• **Description**: A technique that combines a throw with a subsequent joint lock for control after a successful throw.

Execution: Execute a throw (like O Soto Gari) and immediately transition into a joint lock (like Kote Gaeshi) as the opponent falls.

6. **Counters and Defensive Techniques**

Kaeshi Waza (Counter Techniques):

• **Description**: Techniques designed to counter an opponent's attacks effectively.

Execution: Learn to recognize common strikes and transitions into counters, such as executing a throw in response to an incoming strike.

Sutemi Waza (Sacrifice Techniques):

• **Description**: Techniques where the practitioner sacrifices their position to execute a throw or lock.

Execution: Use body weight and timing to create openings, allowing the practitioner to throw the opponent while falling.

Advanced techniques and variations in Shorinji Kempo enhance a practitioner's ability to adapt and respond in various combat scenarios. By mastering these techniques, practitioners develop a deeper understanding of movement, timing, and control, ultimately improving their effectiveness in both training and real-world applications. Regular practice of advanced techniques fosters confidence, skill, and versatility, allowing practitioners to excel in their martial arts journey.

CHAPTER 3: KATA AND FORMS
The Importance Of Kata In Shorinji Kempo

Kata, or pre-arranged forms, hold significant importance in Shorinji Kempo, serving as a vital aspect of training and skill development. These structured sequences of movements encapsulate the principles, techniques, and philosophies of the martial art, providing practitioners with a comprehensive framework for learning and mastery. Here's a detailed look at the importance of kata in Shorinji Kempo:

1. Foundation of Technique:

- **Skill Development**: Kata allows practitioners to practice fundamental techniques (kihon) in a structured manner, enabling them to refine their strikes, kicks, throws, and grappling moves.

• **Muscle Memory**: Repeated practice of kata helps build muscle memory, allowing techniques to be executed with precision and fluidity during sparring or self-defense situations.

2. Understanding Movement:

• **Body Mechanics**: Kata emphasizes proper body mechanics and movement. Practitioners learn to use their hips, feet, and core effectively, which is crucial for generating power and maintaining balance.

• **Footwork and Stances**: Each kata incorporates specific stances (dachi) and footwork, helping practitioners understand the significance of positioning in combat.

3. Application of Techniques:

• **Combining Techniques**: Kata integrates various techniques, demonstrating how to transition smoothly from one move to another. This aids practitioners in understanding the flow of combat and the interconnectedness of techniques.

• **Real-World Scenarios**: While kata is a stylized practice, the movements can be applied to real-world self-defense situations. Practitioners learn to visualize and adapt techniques to different scenarios.

4. Mental Discipline:

• **Focus and Concentration**: Practicing kata requires concentration and mental engagement. This discipline enhances a practitioner's focus, which is essential in both training and combat situations.

• **Mind-Body Connection**: Kata fosters a strong mind-body connection, promoting awareness of one's own movements and the ability to react appropriately to external stimuli.

5. Cultural and Historical Significance:

• **Tradition**: Kata is deeply rooted in the history of Shorinji Kempo and other martial arts. Practicing kata helps preserve the traditions and philosophies passed down through generations.

• **Connection to Philosophy**: Many kata embody the underlying principles of Shorinji Kempo, such as the importance of compassion, respect, and humility. Practitioners internalize these values through kata practice.

6. Assessment and Progression:

• **Belt Promotion**: Kata is often a requirement for belt promotions in Shorinji Kempo. Mastery of specific kata demonstrates a practitioner's understanding and proficiency in the art.

• **Evaluation of Skills**: Instructors assess a student's skills, technique, and understanding of the art through their performance of kata. This evaluation helps identify areas for improvement and guides further training.

7. Building Community and Camaraderie:

• **Group Practice**: Kata can be practiced individually or in groups, fostering a sense of community among practitioners. Group training sessions enhance motivation and support.

• **Shared Goals**: Working on kata together helps create a shared experience among students and instructors, promoting teamwork and camaraderie within the dojo.

Kata plays a crucial role in the practice of Shorinji Kempo, serving as a foundation for technique, mental discipline, and cultural appreciation. Through the study of kata, practitioners develop not only their physical abilities but also their understanding of the philosophy and principles underlying the martial art. Regular practice of kata enhances a practitioner's skill set, mental acuity, and sense of community, making it an indispensable component of Shorinji Kempo training.

Detailed Breakdown Of Key Kata

In Shorinji Kempo, kata are essential for developing skills, understanding techniques, and embodying the philosophy of the martial art. Each kata consists of a series of movements that practitioners perform in a specific order, emphasizing technique, precision, and timing. Below is a detailed breakdown of key kata commonly practiced in Shorinji Kempo:

1. Shoden Kata (Beginner Kata)

Kata 1: Sōke:

• **Overview**: Sōke is often the first kata learned by beginners, introducing fundamental techniques and movements.

Key Techniques:

• Basic stances (zenkutsu dachi, kokutsu dachi)

• Simple punches (oi zuki, gyaku zuki)

• Basic blocks (age uke, gedan barai)

Focus: Emphasis on proper stance, footwork, and basic strikes. Practitioners learn to combine techniques fluidly while maintaining balance.

Kata 2: Henso

• **Overview**: Henso builds on the techniques learned in Sōke, incorporating more complex movements and combinations.

Key Techniques:

• Advanced blocks and strikes (uchi uke, yoko zuki)

• Introduction to kicks (mae geri)

• Basic grappling movements (uchikomi)

Focus: Learning to transition between techniques and applying timing and distance management.

2. Chuden Kata (Intermediate Kata)

Kata 3: Uke

• **Overview**: Uke emphasizes defensive techniques and counters, teaching practitioners to respond effectively to attacks.

Key Techniques:

• Defensive movements (shuto uke, jodan uke)

• Counterattacks (kaeshi zuki)

Introduction to joint locks (kansetsu waza)

Focus: Understanding the importance of timing and leverage while focusing on both defense and counter-offense.

Kata 4: Nage:

• **Overview**: Nage introduces throwing techniques, teaching practitioners to utilize balance and weight distribution.

Key Techniques:

• Various throws (hip throws, shoulder throws)

• Takedowns and sweeps

• Application of kuzushi (breaking balance)

Focus: Emphasizing proper body mechanics, timing, and the relationship between attacker and defender.

3. Juden Kata (Advanced Kata)

Kata 5: Osaekomi:

• **Overview**: Osaekomi focuses on grappling and pinning techniques, teaching practitioners to control opponents effectively.

Key Techniques:

• Various holds and pins (kesa gatame, yoko shiho gatame)

• Joint locks and submissions (ude garami)

• Transitions from standing to ground techniques

Focus: Practitioners learn to maintain control and apply pressure while transitioning between different grappling techniques.

Kata 6: Geri:

• **Overview**: Geri emphasizes advanced kicking techniques, focusing on speed, precision, and combinations.

Key Techniques:

• High kicks (jodan geri, mawashi geri)

• Combination kicks and strikes

• Targeting techniques

Focus: Practitioners refine their kicking techniques, learning to combine them with other strikes and defensive movements.

4. Mastery Kata

Kata 7: Shinjitsu:

• **Overview**: Shinjitsu is often considered a mastery kata, integrating various techniques learned throughout training.

Key Techniques:

• A mix of strikes, kicks, throws, and grappling

• Application of principles learned in previous kata

• Flow and adaptability during performance

Focus: Practitioners work on executing movements fluidly while embodying the principles of Shorinji Kempo, including focus, balance, and self-awareness.

Key Aspects of Kata Practice:

• **Repetition**: Regular practice of kata is essential for skill development and muscle memory. Practitioners should strive for precision and clarity in each movement.

• **Visualization**: Practicing kata involves visualizing an opponent, helping practitioners learn to anticipate and react to attacks.

• **Mindfulness**: Kata practice encourages mindfulness, allowing practitioners to connect their mind and body, promoting a deeper understanding of techniques.

- **Self-Reflection**: After performing kata, practitioners should reflect on their execution, identifying areas for improvement and setting goals for their training.

The detailed breakdown of key kata in Shorinji Kempo provides practitioners with a structured approach to learning and mastering essential techniques. Each kata builds upon previous skills, allowing for gradual progression in both technical proficiency and understanding of the martial art's philosophy.

Regular practice of these kata not only enhances physical abilities but also fosters mental discipline, focus, and a deeper connection to the art of Shorinji Kempo.

Application Of Kata In Sparring

The application of kata in sparring is a crucial aspect of martial arts training, including Shorinji Kempo. While kata consists of pre-arranged movements designed for solo practice, its principles and techniques can be effectively translated into dynamic sparring scenarios. Here's an overview of how kata is applied in sparring and the benefits it offers to practitioners:

1. Translating Techniques from Kata to Sparring:

• **Fundamental Techniques**: The techniques practiced in kata serve as the foundation for movements used in sparring. Practitioners can draw on the strikes, blocks, and footwork learned in kata to respond to live opponents.

- **Combining Movements**: Kata often includes combinations of techniques. In sparring, practitioners can use these combinations to create effective offensive and defensive strategies.

2. Understanding Timing and Distance:

- **Timing**: Kata emphasizes the importance of timing in executing techniques. Practicing kata helps develop an innate sense of timing that practitioners can apply during sparring, allowing them to anticipate and react to their opponent's movements.

- **Distance Management**: Many kata incorporate footwork that teaches practitioners how to control distance. Understanding when to advance, retreat, or close the gap is crucial in sparring scenarios.

3. Defensive Strategies:

• **Blocking and Countering**: Kata often includes defensive techniques such as blocks and counters. Practitioners can apply these techniques during sparring to defend against attacks while setting up their counters.

• **Awareness of Angles**: Many kata teach the importance of angles in both offensive and defensive movements. This awareness can be crucial in sparring, allowing practitioners to evade attacks effectively.

4. Fluidity and Adaptability:

• **Flowing Movements**: Kata promotes smooth transitions between techniques. In sparring, practitioners must adapt to changing circumstances, and the fluidity developed through kata can enhance their ability to flow between techniques seamlessly.

• **Adapting Techniques**: While kata teaches specific movements, sparring often requires adaptability. Practitioners learn to modify techniques based on the opponent's actions and reactions, which is a skill developed through consistent kata practice.

5. Mental Focus and Strategy:

• **Concentration**: The practice of kata requires mental focus and discipline. In sparring, this concentration is vital for maintaining awareness of the opponent and executing techniques effectively.

• **Strategic Thinking**: Practicing kata encourages practitioners to think strategically about movements. In sparring, this mindset enables them to assess the situation and make quick decisions based on the opponent's behavior.

6. Building Confidence and Composure:

• **Confidence in Techniques**: Regular kata practice helps practitioners develop confidence in their abilities. This confidence translates into sparring, allowing them to execute techniques without hesitation.

• **Composure Under Pressure**: The rhythmic nature of kata helps practitioners remain composed under pressure, a valuable trait during sparring where unexpected situations can arise.

7. Integrating Sparring into Kata Practice:

• **Kata in Pairs**: Practicing kata in pairs (known as "kata kumite") allows practitioners to apply the techniques in a controlled sparring environment. This method reinforces the application of kata while fostering teamwork and communication.

• **Sparring Drills**: Incorporating drills that emphasize specific kata techniques during sparring can help practitioners focus on applying learned movements in a live context. This approach reinforces the connection between kata and real combat situations.

8. Feedback and Reflection:

• **Self-Assessment**: After sparring, practitioners can reflect on how effectively they applied kata techniques. This self-assessment helps identify areas for improvement and informs future kata practice.

• **Instructor Feedback**: Instructors can provide feedback on how well students integrate kata techniques into sparring, offering guidance on adjustments and enhancements.

The application of kata in sparring is essential for developing a well-rounded martial artist. By translating the principles and techniques of kata into live sparring scenarios, practitioners enhance their skills in timing, distance management, defense, and adaptability.

Regular practice of kata not only strengthens physical abilities but also fosters mental focus and strategic thinking, leading to greater effectiveness in sparring and self-defense situations.

CHAPTER 4: SPARRING AND APPLICATIONS

Types Of Sparring (Jiyu Kumite)

In Shorinji Kempo, as well as in many martial arts, sparring (known as **jiyu kumite**) plays a vital role in developing practical application skills, timing, and adaptability in real combat scenarios. Different types of sparring offer varied experiences, allowing practitioners to focus on specific aspects of their training. Here's an overview of the main types of sparring in Shorinji Kempo:

1. Jiyu Kumite (Free Sparring):

• **Overview**: Jiyu kumite is the most common form of sparring, allowing practitioners to engage in unscripted combat scenarios. This type of sparring enables fighters to apply techniques learned in kata in a dynamic setting.

Characteristics:

• **Rules**: Sparring can have specific rules regarding allowed techniques, contact levels, and target areas, which vary based on the dojo or competition.

• **Strategy**: Practitioners must use strategy, adaptability, and quick decision-making to respond to their opponent's actions.

• **Environment**: Usually takes place in a controlled environment, such as a dojo or mat area, where safety measures are implemented.

2. Kumite (Point Sparring):

• **Overview**: Kumite, or point sparring, focuses on scoring points for controlled strikes and techniques. The emphasis is on technique and precision rather than full-contact fighting.

Characteristics:

• **Scoring System**: Points are awarded for successfully landing strikes on target areas, typically using specific scoring criteria (e.g., control, technique, and contact).

• **Control**: Practitioners must demonstrate control to prevent excessive force, ensuring the safety of both participants.

• **Competition**: Often used in tournaments, kumite helps practitioners refine their skills under competitive conditions.

3. Grappling Sparring (Ne Waza):

• **Overview**: Grappling sparring focuses on ground techniques, including joint locks, holds, and submissions. This form of sparring is crucial for developing skills in clinch work and ground fighting.

Characteristics:

• **Techniques**: Practitioners apply grappling techniques learned in kata, such as throws and holds, in a live context.

• **Positioning**: Emphasizes positional control, balance, and leverage, allowing practitioners to understand the dynamics of grappling.

• **Integration**: Grappling sparring can be integrated into jiyu kumite to provide a well-rounded approach to combat.

4. Kumite with Specific Techniques:

• **Overview**: This type of sparring involves practitioners focusing on specific techniques or strategies, such as strikes, kicks, or grappling.

Characteristics:

• **Focused Drills**: Participants may engage in drills that emphasize specific movements, such as only using kicks or only employing joint locks.

• **Situational Sparring**: Practitioners may set up specific scenarios (e.g., defending against a punch) to practice targeted responses.

• **Development of Skills**: This method allows for focused improvement on particular techniques while still engaging in a sparring environment.

5. Controlled Sparring (Sparing with Modifications):

• **Overview**: Controlled sparring involves modifying the rules or parameters of sparring to focus on specific skills or to accommodate practitioners of different skill levels.

Characteristics:

• **Restrictions**: Some techniques may be restricted (e.g., no striking to the head) to ensure safety and foster a learning environment.

• **Gradual Introduction**: This type of sparring can help beginners gain confidence before moving on to more intense jiyu kumite.

• **Skill Development**: Practitioners can work on particular areas for improvement, such as timing, distance, or defensive strategies.

6. Sparring with Protective Gear:

• **Overview**: This form of sparring involves practitioners wearing protective gear to allow for a higher intensity of contact while ensuring safety.

Characteristics:

• **Equipment**: Practitioners wear gloves, headgear, shin guards, and other protective equipment.

• **Intensity**: Enables participants to engage more aggressively while minimizing the risk of injury.

• **Realistic Application**: Provides a more realistic experience of combat, preparing practitioners for potential self-defense situations.

7. Sparring in Pair Work:

• **Overview**: Pair work involves two practitioners working together to apply techniques learned in kata and drills in a controlled setting.

Characteristics:

• **Structured Practice**: Allows for a structured approach to practicing specific techniques, such as counters, throws, or joint locks.

• **Feedback**: Partners can provide immediate feedback to each other, enhancing learning and understanding.

- **Adaptability**: Practitioners learn to adapt techniques based on their partner's movements and reactions.

The various types of sparring in Shorinji Kempo provide practitioners with diverse opportunities to apply techniques, develop skills, and enhance their understanding of combat dynamics. By engaging in different sparring formats, students can refine their abilities, gain experience under varying conditions, and build confidence in their martial arts journey. Each type of sparring contributes to the holistic development of a well-rounded martial artist, enabling them to effectively apply their skills in real-life situations.

Sparring Techniques And Strategies

Sparring techniques and strategies are essential for success in Shorinji Kempo and other martial arts. Effective sparring combines technical proficiency, tactical thinking, and adaptability. Here's a comprehensive look at various techniques and strategies that practitioners can utilize during sparring:

Sparring Techniques

1. Striking Techniques

Punches (Tsuki):

• **Jab**: A quick, straight punch used to gauge distance and create openings.

• **Cross**: A powerful straight punch aimed at the opponent's head or body, often following a jab.

• **Hook**: A semi-circular punch targeting the side of the opponent's head or body, effective at close range.

Kicks (Geri):

• **Front Kick (Mae Geri)**: A direct kick to the opponent's body or head, useful for maintaining distance.

• **Roundhouse Kick (Mawashi Geri)**: A powerful kick aimed at the opponent's side or head, using the shin or instep for contact.

• **Side Kick (Yoko Geri)**: A lateral kick that targets the opponent's midsection or legs, effective for disrupting their balance.

Elbows and Knees:

• **Elbow Strikes**: Powerful strikes from close range that can be used when within grappling range.

- **Knee Strikes**: Effective for close combat, targeting the opponent's body or head.

2. Defensive Techniques:

Blocking (Uke):

- **High Block (Jodan Uke)**: Protects the head from overhead strikes.

- **Low Block (Gedan Barai)**: Deflects attacks aimed at the lower body.

- **Parrying**: Redirecting an opponent's strike to create openings for counterattacks.

- **Evasion**: Using footwork and body movement to avoid strikes, such as slipping or ducking under punches.

3. Grappling Techniques

Throws (Nage):

• **Hip Throws (O Goshi)**: Utilizing the hip to throw an opponent off balance.

• **Shoulder Throws (Seoi Nage)**: Leveraging the opponent's weight to execute a throw.

• **Joint Locks (Kansetsu Waza)**: Techniques that control an opponent by manipulating their joints.

• **Takedowns**: Techniques aimed at bringing an opponent to the ground safely and effectively.

<u>**Sparring Strategies**</u>

1. Distance Management:

• **Maintain Distance**: Keeping the right distance allows you to evade strikes while being able to launch your own.

• **Close the Distance**: Understanding when to close the gap to initiate strikes or grappling techniques effectively.

2. Timing and Rhythm

• **Observe Opponent's Timing**: Recognizing patterns in your opponent's movements to anticipate their attacks.

• **Create Opportunities**: Using feints and misdirection to draw reactions from your opponent, creating openings for your strikes.

3. Footwork

• **Mobility**: Staying light on your feet allows you to move in and out of range quickly.

• **Angle Movement**: Moving at angles instead of directly forward or backward to create advantageous positions.

4. Combination Techniques:

• **Set Up Combinations**: Using multiple strikes in succession (e.g., jab-cross-hook) to overwhelm your opponent.

• **Mix Techniques**: Combining strikes, kicks, and grappling techniques to keep your opponent guessing and off-balance.

5. Mindset and Focus:

• **Stay Calm Under Pressure**: Maintaining composure allows you to think clearly and react appropriately.

- **Adaptability**: Being ready to change your strategy based on your opponent's actions and adapting to the flow of the sparring session.

6. Reading Your Opponent:

• **Body Language**: Paying attention to your opponent's posture and movements can provide clues about their intentions.

• **Predicting Actions**: Anticipating what your opponent is likely to do next based on their previous actions.

7. Controlled Aggression:

• **Use of Power**: Knowing when to use power and when to control the intensity, especially in practice settings to ensure safety.

- **Effective Pressure**: Applying pressure without overcommitting, allowing for counterattacks and openings.

Sparring techniques and strategies are essential for developing effective combat skills in Shorinji Kempo. Practitioners should focus on integrating striking, defensive, and grappling techniques while employing strategies centered on distance management, timing, and adaptability.

By refining these skills and strategies, martial artists can enhance their effectiveness in sparring and real-life self-defense situations, ultimately leading to greater proficiency in their martial arts journey. Regular practice and engagement in sparring scenarios will contribute to continuous improvement and deeper understanding of the art.

CHAPTER 5: TRAINING METHODS AND ROUTINES
Warm-Up And Conditioning Exercises

Warm-up and conditioning exercises are crucial components of any martial arts training, including Shorinji Kempo. They help prepare the body for physical activity, reduce the risk of injury, and enhance overall performance. Below is a guide to effective warm-up and conditioning exercises tailored for martial artists.

Warm-Up Exercises: A proper warm-up should gradually increase the heart rate and loosen the muscles, joints, and tendons. Here are some effective warm-up exercises:

1. Dynamic Stretching:

• **Leg Swings**: Swing one leg forward and backward while holding onto a wall for balance. Perform 10-15 swings per leg to loosen the hip flexors.

• **Arm Circles**: Extend your arms to the sides and make small circles, gradually increasing the size. Do this for about 30 seconds in each direction.

• **Torso Twists**: Stand with feet shoulder-width apart and twist your torso side to side, keeping your hips facing forward. Perform 10-15 twists on each side.

2. Cardiovascular Warm-Up:

• **Jumping Jacks**: Perform 30 seconds of jumping jacks to elevate the heart rate and increase circulation.

• **High Knees**: Jog in place, bringing your knees up towards your chest. Do this for 30 seconds.

• **Butt Kicks**: Jog in place while kicking your heels towards your glutes. Perform this for 30 seconds.

3. Joint Rotations:

• **Neck Rolls**: Gently roll your head in a circular motion to loosen the neck. Perform 5 rolls in each direction.

• **Wrist and Ankle Rolls**: Rotate each wrist and ankle clockwise and counterclockwise for about 10 rotations in each direction.

4. Movement Drills:

• **Shadow Fighting**: Practice your basic techniques (strikes, kicks, blocks) in the air, focusing on form and fluidity. Spend about 2-3 minutes on this.

• **Footwork Drills**: Move around the training area, practicing advancing, retreating, and lateral movements. Incorporate stances like zenkutsu dachi and kokutsu dachi.

Conditioning Exercises

Conditioning exercises build strength, endurance, flexibility, and overall fitness, all of which are essential for martial arts performance. Here are some effective conditioning exercises:

1. Strength Training:

• **Push-Ups**: A fundamental exercise that builds upper body strength. Aim for 3 sets of 10-15 repetitions.

• **Squats**: A great exercise for building leg strength and stability. Perform 3 sets of 15-20 repetitions.

- **Planks**: Strengthens the core. Hold a plank position for 30-60 seconds, repeating 2-3 times.

2. Plyometrics:

- **Jump Squats**: Perform a squat and explode into a jump, landing softly and returning to the squat position. Do 3 sets of 10-12 repetitions.

- **Burpees**: Combine a squat, push-up, and jump into one fluid movement. Perform 3 sets of 5-10 repetitions.

3. Cardiovascular Conditioning:

- **Interval Training**: Engage in short bursts of high-intensity activity (e.g., sprinting) followed by periods of rest or low-intensity activity. For example, sprint for 30 seconds, then walk for 1 minute. Repeat for 15-20 minutes.

• **Circuit Training**: Combine several exercises (e.g., jumping jacks, push-ups, lunges, and mountain climbers) in a circuit format, performing each for 30 seconds with minimal rest.

4. Flexibility and Mobility:

• **Static Stretching**: After the workout, hold stretches for major muscle groups (hamstrings, quadriceps, shoulders) for 15-30 seconds to enhance flexibility.

• **Yoga or Tai Chi**: Incorporate practices that focus on flexibility, balance, and body awareness, which can be beneficial for martial artists.

A well-structured warm-up and conditioning routine is essential for effective training in Shorinji Kempo. Incorporating dynamic stretching, cardiovascular exercises, and strength training helps prepare the body for the demands of martial arts, improves performance, and reduces the risk of injury. Practicing these exercises regularly will enhance your overall fitness and effectiveness in sparring and kata, leading to a more rewarding martial arts journey.

Conclusion

Engaging in Shorinji Kempo offers a holistic approach to martial arts, encompassing physical, mental, and spiritual development. From the foundational techniques and principles to the various sparring methods and conditioning routines, each aspect of training plays a vital role in shaping a well-rounded martial artist.

The practice of warm-up and conditioning exercises prepares practitioners not only to perform at their best but also to prevent injuries, ensuring longevity in their training.

Sparring techniques and strategies encourage adaptability, quick thinking, and the application of learned skills in dynamic environments, fostering both confidence and competence.

Moreover, the philosophical and ethical dimensions of Shorinji Kempo instill values of respect, discipline, and perseverance, reinforcing the importance of character development alongside physical prowess. As practitioners immerse themselves in this rich martial art, they cultivate not only their fighting abilities but also a deeper understanding of themselves and their place within the larger community.

Ultimately, the journey through Shorinji Kempo is not just about mastering techniques; it is about personal growth, building connections with others, and embodying the principles of balance, harmony, and resilience in every aspect of life. Whether you are a beginner or an experienced martial artist, the continuous exploration of Shorinji Kempo promises to enhance both your physical capabilities and your life beyond the dojo.

Glossary Of Terms

Here's a glossary of terms commonly used in Shorinji Kempo and martial arts in general. This list can serve as a valuable reference for practitioners and those interested in learning about the art.

- **Atemi**: Striking techniques aimed at sensitive points on the body.
- **Atemi Waza**: Techniques specifically designed for striking.
- **Bunkai**: The application or interpretation of kata movements in real combat scenarios.

- **Bokken**: A wooden training sword used for practicing techniques.
- **Chudan**: The middle level; a position or strike targeting the torso or midsection.
- **Combat**: Engaging in a physical fight or sparring with an opponent.
- **Dachi**: Stance or position of the feet, fundamental to martial arts movements.
- **Zenkutsu Dachi**: Front stance.
- **Kokutsu Dachi**: Back stance.
- **Dojo**: Training hall or school where martial arts are practiced.
- **Empi**: Elbow strikes used in close combat.
- **Geri**: Kicking techniques used to strike an opponent.

- **Grappling**: Techniques involving holds, throws, and submissions in close combat.

- **Gyaku Tsuki**: Reverse punch, often used as a powerful striking technique.

- **Hiki Waza**: Techniques involving pulling or drawing an opponent closer.

- **Hiza Geri**: Knee kick, targeting the opponent's midsection or head.

- **Jiyu Kumite**: Free sparring, where practitioners engage in unscripted combat.

- **Jodan**: The upper level; refers to techniques or targets above the waist.

- **Kansetsu Waza**: Joint locking techniques used to control or submit an opponent.

- **Kata**: Pre-arranged patterns of movements practiced solo or in pairs to develop technique and form.

- **Kenshi**: A practitioner of Shorinji Kempo; often translated as "warrior" or "martial artist."

- **Mawashi Geri**: Roundhouse kick, targeting the side of an opponent.

- **Mu**: A state of emptiness or stillness, often referenced in meditation and practice.

- **Nage**: Throwing techniques used to bring an opponent to the ground.

- **Osaekomi**: Pinning techniques used to control an opponent on the ground.

- **Rei**: Bowing; a sign of respect in martial arts practice and rituals.

- **Renzoku**: Continuous techniques or movements performed in succession.

- **Sparring**: Practicing fighting techniques against an opponent in a controlled environment.

- **Shorinji Kempo**: A modern martial art that combines self-defense, physical fitness, and spiritual development.

- **Tsuki**: Striking techniques, particularly punches.

- **Tachi**: A term for standing techniques or stances.

- **Tachi Waza**: Standing techniques used in grappling.

- **Uke**: A receiver of techniques, typically the person being attacked or the one practicing defenses.

- **Ushiro**: Referring to the back; often used in context to movements or techniques.

- **Yoko Geri**: Side kick, targeting an opponent's midsection or head from the side.

- **Yudansha**: A practitioner who has attained a black belt rank.

The purpose of this glossary is to provide a foundational understanding of core concepts that are associated with Shorinji Kempo and martial arts. By becoming familiar with these phrases, one can improve their ability to communicate during training, increase their level of grasp of techniques, and boost their entire learning experience.

Kameron Jalen, an author, frequently employs his profound comprehension of human nature and personal experiences to investigate a diverse array of themes in his writing. His compositions may encompass instructional materials, non-fiction, or fiction, which demonstrate his capacity to articulate intricate concepts in a manner that is both engaging and comprehensible. Jalen's objective in his writing is to motivate and inspire readers by imparting knowledge on the significance of personal development, self-discipline, and resilience.

Kameron Jalen is also a dedicated martial arts practitioner, having trained in a variety of disciplines. His proficiency in martial arts is not only indicative of his physical abilities, but also underscores the philosophical and cerebral components of the discipline. He is likely to promote the advantages of martial arts in the development of focus, discipline, and confidence, and he may conduct seminars or teach classes to disseminate his expertise. He integrates the principles of hard work and perseverance into both his writing and teaching, as evidenced by his martial arts journey.

Kameron Jalen has a Ph.D. in a pertinent discipline from a prestigious university in the United States, in addition to his creative and physical activities. His academic education equips him with a robust foundation for his writing and teaching, enabling him to approach subjects with a critical and analytical perspective. His scholarly work and research may concentrate on the social implications of martial arts, human behavior, or psychology, thereby contributing to both academic discourse and practical applications.

Kameron Jalen possesses an uncommon combination of academic rigor, physical prowess, and creativity. He remains a source of inspiration and influence for those in his vicinity, motivating them to pursue their interests and aspire for excellence in all aspects of life because of his diverse talents. Jalen is dedicated to the promotion of personal and professional development, whether through his academic lectures, martial arts classes, or publications.

THE END